Just How Well Do You Know Your Body

ISBN: 1-4196-3575-1
Library of Congress Control Number : 2006903574

To order additional copies, please contact us.
BookSurge, LLC
www.booksurge.com
1-866-308-6235
orders@booksurge.com

BRENDA
SUTTON

JUST HOW WELL
DO YOU KNOW
YOUR BODY

2006

Just How Well Do You Know Your Body

A Big thanks to the following:

My Dad: Thanks for all you love and support throughout my life. I Love You!!!!!!!!

My Mom: Thanks for always being there as my mom and best friend. I Love You!!!!!!

My Brother: Thank you for all your love and support. I Love You!!!!!

My Step Father: Thank you for all you have done and accepting my brother and I as one of your own children. I Love You!!!!!!!

My Ex-Husband: Thanks for always supporting me in my decisions and being there and never looking at me any different`.

My Boss: What can I say?????Thanks for listening and being there for all my ups and downs.

My family: You all are so great and understanding and I Love You All!!!!!

My Church Family: Thank you for all the prayers during all my surgeries.

A Big Thanks To:
Dr. Elizabeth Pritchard
Dr. Jack Sanford and staff
Dr. Robert Wallace

Catherine Stroud Martin: You are my Circle of Life! You have been there for me as my doctor and friend. You always believed in me , never judged me and have always found what is wrong with me health wise. You were there when I felt like my life was falling apart and now we are fighting lupus and bladder and health together. Thank you for everything you do and have done for me for the past ten or fifteen years. You are an angel in everyway. I Love You!!!!!

The staff with the UT Medical Group
You all are my angels in White!!!!!!!!!

*In loving memory of the following who have touched my life
in many ways:*

Mary Cubine
Scotty Dunavant
Thomas Burns Johnson
Clara Shands
Eunice Sutton
Oma Troublefield
Barry White

WOMEN, DO YOU KNOW YOUR BODIES??

We never want to think that anything can go wrong in our perfect world, that we will always be happy and healthy, and have the perfect life. Wake up!!!! That is in a perfect world and WE do not live in one!!

We all go through our daily routines, get up, get ready for work, come home, and do all we have to do before bed. We, as women, give and give sometimes ignoring ourselves. We, as wives, mothers, and partners, as WOMEN, deserve more than we allow ourselves.

Now get this: I'm not talking about money or anything extravagant. I'm saying, "Just how well do you actually know your body?"

I never understood all of the yearly pap smears, breast exams, and hormone changes—and everything that goes along with these changes. From hot flashes, to weight fluctuation, to hair falling out so it's so thin you can see your scalp when it's wet. Heck, sometimes you can even see your scalp when it's not wet and you wonder.... If this is what it's like in my 40's what's it going to be like at 50, 60, and so on?

I'm not a writer nor have I done anything that great in my life, but as a woman, I have survived more than I ever could imagine, all because I took notice of myself and my body. I thank God everyday for helping me to realize that I do not live in that perfect world we all hope for.

I have had so many pap smears my gynecologist can tell

who I am without seeing my face. I have had so many female surgeries that I would draw on my tummy for a joke so that when I was put to sleep at least someone would get a laugh.

I can remember being in grade school and telling my mom one morning that my stomach hurt. With all the love and support from my mother she told me, "go on to school and if you do not feel better call and I will come and get you." I was in the auditorium, the bell rang for class, and down the steps I went, no really, DOWN the steps I went. The next thing I remember was the principal and a teacher standing over me saying, "Get up" and I was scared and wanted my mom. They got me up, my side was killing me (at least I thought it was actually going to kill me) and they said, "Do you think you can go to class?" With mule tears (not to be confused with crocodile tears) I said, "Call my mom." She came and got me. A few hours later I woke up in the hospital with a cut on my stomach and pain. That's when I learned to listen to my body. I believe I was about 11 or 12 years old, and that was my first female surgery. No one can imagine that just being a female can cause so much drama; Eve should have left that dang apple alone. Eve never had the chance to have female trouble; all she had was a BIG appetite.

Every month, all I could think about was the cramps coming again. Just like clockwork, the cramps would come, the cravings and the flooding. My mood was like the "she-devil." NOW, I know that if I don't take the hormones, I AM the "she-devil." Have you ever thought about slapping your spouse because he just wanted to watch ESPN? Or maybe find a football and pay someone to tackle him to just get pleasure out of it? I only felt that way when it was time for the good ole hormone shot. Do you feel me yet? Let's go on.

Okay, let me back up a few years, before the hormone

shots or the husband. From ages 12 to 18, I never knew when my period was coming or even if it would. Sometimes when it came, it would last the normal seven days or sometimes it would last the whole month. I should have bought into a blood bank. Just kidding. My mom would take me back and forth to the ob-gyn; that's why he could tell who I was so easy. Anyway, we tried everything. I had so many ultrasounds from abdominal to vaginal. At 13, I felt like I was being violated. If I had one now, being over 40 and divorced, the vaginal ultrasound might be enjoyable, if it didn't cost $1,000 or more. Again, I'm just kidding. So here I am young and dumb, being violated (okay, seems like) several times a month, pap smear after pap smear. The blue junk they put on our vaginas, because of the antibiotics, has caused a yeast infection, and turns our cute bikini panties (before thongs, remember) blue in the crotch. So here we stand, all pissed off again, because that blue stuff is there forever and a day and my cute panties are ruined.

When the ultrasound results come in, the phone rings. They have scheduled surgery again. At least you get to sleep and afterwards they give you drugs for the pain. The gas they use for laparoscopic surgery, whew, all you want to do is toot. When it finally comes to the tooting it's a great big fart and boy oh boy do you feel better. As women, we rarely fart, right? When I expelled the gas they used, I just prayed no one was in harm's way.

Lets see; now I am about 16 or 17 and they want to take out one ovary and tube. No big deal, right? Wrong!!!! Understand, I have probably already been through over 30 surgeries to "save" my female organs; now they want to take out one whole set. Here I am in the hospital the night before surgery and they bring in this gigantic bag filled with fluid. I'm wondering, what the crap does this nurse think she is going to do with this thing and she's gonna put it WHERE??? I figured it out real quick; I almost broke my neck running to the restroom. That's where the real fun began. Here I am, in all my glory, hoping (no, praying) no one is coming to visit me in the hospital the night before they go in and take out part of my baby makers. After I was finally finished in the restroom, the nurse comes back in the room with a razor and a prep kit to take care of the hair problem and then hands me ANOTHER bag filled with fluid. All I could think about was, I know she doesn't think I have anything left in my tummy. Everything I had in my stomach had been flushed to China by now. I turned to my mom with this crazy look and she assured me this time the bag was for something else, BOY, was I relieved. There was a part of me that was really scared to go back into the restroom, because that bag sure looked like the other one. I knew my body well enough to know that it could NOT take another enema!

Now here I am, shaved, emptied out, and the bag is still hanging over the toilet. I ask my mom what does she want me to do with this one? Lucky me, I found out what a douche is. Now, I have been cleaned out, emptied out, shaved down like a baby, and disinfected. What in the world is next? By this time, I am physically exhausted. There's a knock on the door to my hospital room, it's "that" nurse again and she's bringing me this little foil package of Neosporin. All I could think of is, what is this for? She hands me the Neosporin and tells me to put this on, nothing else. I go into the bathroom—my mom is thinking I know what to do—and proceeded to try and get all that Neosporin inside me. In my mind, everything else went up there, so why not this? After a grueling 30 minutes, my mom asks me, "Are you okay?" I came out of the restroom and told her I had trouble getting that up inside me. She laughed and said, "it's not suppose to go up there, you were suppose to rub it on where they shaved you so you won't itch and get razor bumps." I felt so stupid! But we both got a big laugh out of it.

The day of the surgery, all I remember is waking up wanting my panties on. I thought I would get to lay in the bed and actually sleep off all the medication, but about 6:30 p.m. the nurse, yeah the same one from the night before, comes in and says let's go for a walk. I looked at her like she has lost every bit of sense God gave her. She gets me out of bed to walk and I could not straighten my torso up to normal. I looked like an old lady trying to walk, bent over and shuffling my feet. I got halfway up the hall and I told her I was going back to lie down and to LEAVE ME ALONE. This went on and on for five to seven days until I finally got to go home.

Now lets go on to after what the doctors call a partial hysterectomy and me, I call HELL! It had to be one of the worst surgeries I had ever had or thought I would ever have. Okay, I have one less ovary and one less tube so the other one is supposed to kick in and take up the slack, right? What I found out was, mine did not want to. The job must have been too much for the little guy!!!(In the mood I was in, "guy" seemed appropriate) So the poor little guy only worked when it was convenient for him (still seems appropriate—huh). So that was not always the best thing for me. What was I supposed to do, ground (you know, the punishment our parents give us for doing wrong) my ovary for two weeks because it did not want to always work?

When my ovary did work, it did a good job. When it didn't work it made me feel like crap! My side would hurt and I would have hormone flashes (I really did not know what they were at that time). As the years went on I learned real quick what a hot flash was. When I was younger and having hot flashes, I just thought my parents were too cheap to turn the air conditioner on!

Trying to keep this lazy ovary, so that someday I could have a baby, I went through surgery after surgery removing big cysts, cleaning up endometriosis, and anything else that seemingly could go wrong.

I can remember the look on my parents' faces every time I had to go under the knife. They hurt for me so much. As for me, I thought this was a normal way of life. Since I began my monthly cycle, I thought all women went through what I was going through. I learned that every time my body had a pain, I bled too much; it was a sign that my body was trying to tell me to go back to my ob-gyn. Don't you know he got sick and tired of seeing my butt (okay, maybe not my butt) all the time. I was sick of him looking down there. I hated going, I felt like at my age, why does he have to look down there all the time, or why do I have to drink gallons of water for the ultrasound? As much water as I always had to drink I could have floated to the doctor's office. Heck, Noah didn't see as much water as I drank! So here I was lying on the table for the ultrasound, full of water, and what does the ultrasound tech do, she pushes on my stomach with this "thing" to take pictures of my insides with me having to pee like a racehorse. Does she care??? No, but I bet if I had used the bathroom on her table she would have. That would have been one of those times you could say piss on it, and mean it.

So I'm older now, maybe 19 or so, and my doctor tells me if I want a child I better start thinking about having one. I've been dating this guy for several years and I go home and tell him to come over to talk. I break the news and we think about it for several months. We get engaged and try to get pregnant. Easy, right? Not!

So for several months, we're like rabbits; only one thing came clear to me, I was not getting pregnant. I went back to my doctor and told him that I did as he said, like rabbits, nothing happening. So he gives me a fertility pill and tells me to drink some wine to relax, then afterwards (yes, the rabbit thing) hold my butt in the air for ten minutes or so. Now, you know that can't look very pretty. Well, to make a long story short, we did this for about a year and then I find out he is as much of slime as the crap he was ejaculating. He sure would have made pretty babies, though (if you get my meaning). Now I have a real problem: no baby and no man to help with the process. I know we don't need a man for the process these days, but remember this was in the early 1990's and I was only 20 years old at this point.

We break up, but in the next few months I started having female troubles AGAIN. This time it was really, really (did I mention really) painful. It felt like knives being stuck in my side, my back and anywhere else that could hurt.

I go back to the ob-gyn, and he tells me to think about a complete hysterectomy! WHAT?? I am only 20 years old, never been married or pregnant. What was he thinking? Every woman wants (remember, the 1990's) a loving husband then a family and a house with the white picket fence. Right? To have my doctor tell me this was the craziest thing I had ever heard. I refused to listen and told him no way and left. One thing you need to understand, this man (my doctor) was my lifeline, I trusted him to the utmost, but at that moment he was JUST a MAN and had no idea what I was feeling inside my heart, not my butt (okay, okay, but you know what I mean).

Several weeks went by and I was taking a lot of pain meds,

antibiotics and steroids. Now, before all this started I was four foot eleven inches and about 115 pounds. I am still four foot eleven and about 140 pounds. I was rolling around instead of walking. As long as the meds kept me from hurting so bad I would cry I didn't care. I was still in denial over the complete hysterectomy news. Several more weeks went by and the pain got worse and the weight was now approximately 190 pounds. Can you imagine...? I was as round as I was tall. Things were really going downhill now and I was rolling downhill because I was too big to walk down it.

Now I have this decision to make, and who do most of us turn to when we need to talk and want the right answers, besides GOD? Our mothers, and my mom has always stood beside me, in the hospital and at home. I have cried on her shoulders so many times she is still wearing a raincoat. She probably wishes she had a raincoat and umbrella at times—and earplugs.

At this point in my life my parents had divorced after 25 years of marriage (talk about when it rains it pours, that water again). I had accepted their divorce but this was something I could not accept. My doctor and all the nurses had worked so hard to save my female organs so I could have a child, and now the parts that make you a woman are going to be ripped out of me and thrown away. I felt like no man would ever want to marry me because I was not complete. I had all the love and support from my parents and my brother. We call our family meetings the round table, so here we are "at the round table" again. My family helps me realize that my health is the most important issue and we, as a family, can work through the rest. So the decision is made: I have to go through with the surgery. My mother calls my doctor and now we are going in for the worst appointment of my life, at least I thought it was the end of me being a woman. I believe my faith was really weak at this time in my life.

We all have said, I wish I knew then what I know now; life just does not work that way. Too bad, we all would be so much smarter. I think women as a whole are a lot smarter than most men anyway but opinions are like butt holes: we all have one and they usually stink.

Now I am at the doctor's office to schedule the surgery and my doctor tells me that he knew, in time, I would be back, but it would be on my time. Well, he was right. I was so tired at this point, maybe because of the pain and the weight I was caring around.

Now the time has come for me to check in the hospital again. I am sure that by now I have paid for the west wing of the Baptist Hospital. It's pretty bad when you walk up to the floor for surgery and the nurses say your name and ask how you are doing BEFORE you even get checked in. This time I am a little smarter about all the pre-operation stuff. I get all the pre-op stuff done and they give me a sleeping pill (like that was going to help since I was scared to death) and tell me to get a good night sleep. Yeah, right!

It is morning and time to go into the cold operating room; at least they give me a blanket out of a warmer this time. The nurse tells me to move to the table and put my butt close to the hole that is cut out on the operating table. I asked her what the hole is for and she tells me it's for the doctor to throw instruments and gauze in. I thought when I was put to sleep maybe I would pee and they wanted it to go in a bedpan. Then the anesthesiologist tells me to count backwards from 100, I remember saying 97, now tell me that's not some good stuff they give you. The next thing I remember is waking up in recovery wondering if I had died and gone to hell! The pain was a ten plus ten. The nurse advises me I am on a pump for the pain medication, well I hit that thing but nothing happened. I thought, oh okay, it would just take time. I could hit this pump every three minutes and don't think I missed one minute. The pain was excruciating regardless of how many times I hit that pump. I know my body was hurting and I could not get anyone to listen to me in that recovery room. I was taken back to my room where my family was waiting. I was crying, the pain was so bad. My mom tried to put pillows in areas to relieve the pain, my brother was figuring the times I could hit the pump so it would not run out before time, my daddy was standing at the end of the bed with tears in his eyes. This went on for most of the afternoon and my brother looked at the pump and said "it hasn't moved, she isn't getting anything." I tried to tell them my body was hurting like hell. My brother finally got in touch with my doctor and he came right over; thank goodness his office is just across the street from the hospital. I guess all those years tending me paid off, because he cleaned house (and I don't mean he dusted and vacuumed) with the nurse that was ignoring my screams for help. He ordered a shot, and a new pump ASAP, no not ASAP, but PDQ (pretty damn quick). I finally got some relief after five or six hours of pain. I had moved around on the rough sheets until my elbows were raw. This is when I think nurses need to realize that sometimes the patient understands his or her body better than science does. Don't you think? I have finally gotten comfortable, the best I could be, and this hateful nurse I have had all day wants me to get up and walk. I started yelling ugly things to her and she calls in a psychiatrist because she thinks I'm losing it. When he comes in, without my doctor knowing this, he starts telling me how I am feeling and what he thinks I need to do. I was so angry, I threw a blow dryer at him. Needless to say, he never came back. That afternoon my doctor came in and my mom told him everything that had been going on. He went ballistic! The hateful nurse was reprimanded! She probably felt like she had a new bunghole ripped. Hope it hurt, since she allowed me to hurt for most of the day. I know she had never had surgery or listened to her patients who know their bodies.

I hope if any nurses and doctors are reading this it SHOULD be a lesson; sometimes the patient knows best (it's sorta like that "walk a mile in my shoes" cliché) or at least those patients do that truly know their own bodies. Now, this does NOT mean I don't trust nurses or doctors, just that sometimes in their jobs they forget that every patient is not the same. All I am trying to say is "Listen to your patients."

I was going through so many emotions during my healing process; later in life I found out they are all normal processes. We will get to that. At times, I was feeling like I was the only woman in the world going through HELL! I felt so alone even though I had wonderful, loving support from my family and my doctor.

I had been in the hospital so many times before but this was the only time I felt so bad and overcome with loneliness. I just wasn't myself at all.

Before my hysterectomy, (I forgot this part until now) I was in the hospital for three solid months. This will let you understand more of what I went through up until this point. The reason for such a long stay in the hospital is this: I had started feeling like I was coming down with the flu. I started taking aspirin and regular over-the-counter cold medications. At this point in my life, remember my parents were divorced, my dad was living in my hometown, my mom was living in the next state over and my brother was in college. So, as I was self-medicating the flu symptoms, and my mom would call and check on me I would just say, "I'm fine." Several days went by and I really could not get to feeling any better, and I started my period. The flu is bad, but my period was always as bad as bad can get, if not worse. This went on for about two days and the cramps and flu were really, really, getting me down. I had a fever of 104, sometimes even higher. A good friend came to see me and she took me to the emergency room where they sent me straight to (GUESS WHO) my ob-gyn. My fever now is 105 and I am sicker than sick. My doctor put me straight in the hospital; my fever was so high I went into a light coma. (You know where you can hear everyone talking around you but you can't talk back or wake up.) So, here I am in the bed with a high fever, the doctor and nurses kept packing me in ice. I was receiving strong antibiotics by IV and the doctor is telling my parents there is a possibility that I would have brain damage when and if I did wake up because of my fever being so extremely high. My parents at this point just thought they had been through a tough time with my health, but this tested every type of strength they both had. I don't really remember how long I was out of it, but I did finally come to and did not have any brain damage (though widely disbelieved by some, my brother for one—HA!!) but I did have a terrible infection in my blood and female organs. The doctor was afraid of me getting blood clots, so he started giving me a blood thinner twice a day by shot (oh NO, couldn't be by mouth) in my stomach. Then came radiation, ZAP, ZAP. I know what you are thinking at this point, why would I not want a total hysterectomy? I WANTED A CHILD OF MY OWN! You're thinking I'm selfish now, but really I'm not! I'm just a young woman with the All American dream! So, I had a few more surgeries, finally received the right antibiotics, radiation, and was on the road to recovery from this episode. Thanksgiving passed and so did my birthday and I finally got to go home. My hair had started thinning really bad. I went to the beauty shop to the lady that had always cut my hair, and while she was washing my hair, we were talking, and suddenly she got very quiet. When I asked her, "What's wrong?" she replied, "Don't worry, just so you know, I have been where you are right now. Your hair is falling out." I'm not only getting fat, now you're telling me I may or may not go bald. Of course, I had to realize this was not her fault. We decided to cut my hair real short and I kept it short for a long time. I think I may have left this out earlier, maybe because I did not want to remember. If I'm going to tell you some things, I HAVE to tell you EVERYTHING.

Back to the healing process of the hysterectomy: the doctor comes into my room to tell me that when they went to remove my uterus, cervix, and tube/ovary, every organ was like mush and fell apart. Then I'm told that I would probably never been able to conceive a child anyway (now you KNOW the rabbit stuff and holding my butt in the air had to cross my mind). SO WHAT THE HELL! (Like that eased the pain any, BS)

Facing the fear of having to poop after surgery is awful. If you have ever had surgery you can relate. After being cut open from hipbone to hipbone and your insides thrown around like garbage, pooping is not something you look forward to. Tooting feels good, pooping feels like crap. (No pun intended.) Preparing for a poop should not be a big deal, but during this time you can only pray everything will be soft and not hard. The nurses come in and ask everyday, "Have you had a bowel movement today?"

You want to lie, because you know you can't go home until you poop. When the big day finally comes, even though it hurts like CRAP (pun intended), you are relieved to tell her, "YES!"

Learning to deal with your hormones is another test of strength (or God's sense of humor). The hormones really do a woman's body good. I am going back to the hysterectomy; now the nurse comes in with this little yellow pill (later I realize I will fall in love with this one) called premarin1.25. She tells me I will have to take this once a day from now on. For those of you who still have all of your baby makers, this is for menopause. Someday you all will understand this part. This is where the hot flashes, cold flashes and night sweat come to bear, not including the mood swings. All of this comes to a head after they take out your baby parts, and believe me it does not get any better with age. A few days pass and I tell the nurse, "I don't think that pill is working." She replies, "Give it SIX weeks and see how things go." Now six weeks of all this is BULL. Don't ya think? I knew in six weeks I had to go back to my doctor for a post-op checkup and if my hormones were still driving me to sweat, swear, and everything else, I would tell him.

(At this time I'm stupid on how they check hormone levels.)

I am released from the hospital and on my way to my mother's house so she can help me (Dads aren't that great at all of this, even though they want to help). I arrive at my mother's and lay my big butt (still at least 180 pounds) on her couch praying my butt will not get any wider. I could be watching a beer commercial and start crying. I had to change my gown two or three times a day because of the sweats. Having to shower four or five times a day, screaming at everyone who called or came by.

I was thinking after two weeks at home my hormones would have at least started leveling out some. Wrong! I didn't know what nerves were until now. You have all heard someone say, "You are getting on my last nerve!" Well after a hysterectomy, EVERYBODY gets on your nerves, even the dog.

One day I'm in the shower and look down to wash the incision and it has started busting open, small holes all the way across my scar. I call my mom in the bathroom and she tells me to get dressed she is taking me to the emergency room, something isn't right. When we arrived at the hospital, the nurse takes me right back to a room. The doctor comes in and is amazed that this would happen after three or four weeks. He calls my doctor and tells him what he has found. They come up with: I have healed on the outside but not the inside. Everyone knows you're supposed to heal inside out. Not me, guess I'm not normal. We are told to take Q-tips, dip them in hydrogen peroxide and stick the Q-tips inside each hole in the scar several times a day. Talk about hurt! This was done until my six-week checkup.

Six weeks have passed, time for the checkup. Mother takes me to the doctor yet again, and I tell his nurse all about the symptoms of the hormones. She tells me she can check my levels by a simple blood test. Now why in the world could the nurse in the hospital not have done the same? (Ms Know It All.) I'm put in a room yet again, sitting in a paper gown waiting on the doctor. He comes in, we talk about the hormones, the scar, and he does another pelvic exam. Why? I thought you took everything!

His nurse knocks on the exam room door and she has this HUGE needle. I sit wondering, what in the world is this for? I was told, "here is a hormone shot." She puts this HUGE needle in my hip, this shot was BIG and thick and hurt like hell going in, but the symptoms got better in a few days.

I go back home with my mom and we get a call a few days

later from the doctor's office. It's the nurse and she tells me my hormone levels are ZERO. I couldn't tell whether ZERO is good or bad at this point, but guess what, of course—BAD! Now I have to take a hormone shot once a month along with the hormone pill everyday. I had to learn to give myself the hormone shot in the thigh area. This was not fun; I didn't realize the shots would break down tissue in my thighs. But they did! My skin and muscle tissue are so tough no shot can break the skin now.

Hope you all are still with me and not bored to tears. I'm taking the hormone pill and now this painful shot that is as thick as molasses, what else can go wrong? Bet you are wondering if I am still thunder butt. Not as bad, now I am probably about 145 pounds. I figure if I am not a complete woman on the inside I should at least try and look better on the outside. I am trying really hard to keep my composure and lose the weight. I know I'm too short to be so round. I don't know which is harder at this point: losing the weight or coming to terms with losing all the baby maker parts.

I'm thinking, now everything is fixed and life should just go on. I've already reached the $1 million lifetime benefit with my health insurance (go figure—huh). What do I do? I still owe over $180,000 in medical bills. At the ripe ole age of 22 I have to file bankruptcy. I really felt like a failure. I'd been working since I was 14 years old, going to school, for what? BANKRUPTCY? I knew this was NOT my parent's responsibility. It was mine. So I filed, and I really felt like my life was ruined.

And of course, my life was not ruined. My life was just put on hold with a few disappointments along the way. Women are supposed to always be the strong ones. Men are the ones who have the happy-go-lucky attitudes with absolutely no worries. I say, "Whatever."

I feel like half of a woman and broke. (Not to be confused with being cut in half.) I began having bad headaches (go figure), so I go back to my ob-gyn, thinking this is due to hormones or stress. For once I was right, learning to really listen to my body! I knew headaches were not supposed to be so bad that all you want is a dark, quiet room.

I go to the doctor, who tells me it is probably stress and out-of-whack hormones combined. (GO FIGURE.) He tells me about a new drug that is FDA approved and NON-ADDICTIVE. He gives me a prescription to get filled at my pharmacy for the headaches. I begin taking the medication as instructed by my doctor. It works. But it came at a very high price and I'm not talking about how much the medication cost. Not knowing that the drug was actually ADDICTIVE, even though I was told otherwise, I took this whenever I needed it. Needless to say, I got ADDICTED to a NON-ADDICTIVE medication. If you're asking, "DO WHAT?" no, you're not confused nor are you reading this wrong. The medication was supposed to be so GREAT, NON-ADDICTIVE and, I might add, I wasn't the only person who was misinformed on this medication. This was not the fault of my doctor; he only relayed what he had read concerning the medication. So don't always believe what you read! YOU CAN BELIEVE ALL OF THIS YOU ARE READING! Getting back to the subject: My doctor has prescribed a wonderful drug that helps headaches, but now I get a bigger problem than I ever expected. I AM ADDICTED! How could this happen? I get into trouble (not the kind of trouble you hear about when it comes to girls (see above, get it??)), but at the time I didn't realize what was about to happen. Remember, I was not the only person who had been misinformed about this medication. Around 25 to 30 others had also been misinformed, but we all got our attorney fees paid, if you know what I mean. This is all I am legally able to say about this. (CLASS ACTION, HINT.)

After this point in my life, what else is going to go wrong? I change jobs and become more involved in my church. I had a BIG wakeup call, because, needless to say, I'd lost a lot of my faith, which I have now begun to find again. (Thank God, literally.)

I felt like I'd disappointed my parents, my brother and the rest of my family and friends. I never understood just how strong love from family and friends could be until this point in my life. I know my heart was broken and I'd broken all of their hearts too. I had to make things right, and not only to myself. Silly me just couldn't understand why I was living life the wrong way. I had to get my priorities back in order, so that's exactly what I did.

I am around 30 at this point in my life; I have gotten my family and my faith back in order. Now know this, when I turned 30, I felt like most people do when they turn 40 (I know this because I'm past 40 now). To me, turning 30 was awful and I know it's not my hormones because they are under control. So why did I feel so bad about turning 30?

I still have not met the man of my life (please God, tell me this isn't just a myth from the Dr. Phils of the world) and I'm thinking I'm getting wrinkles, etc., but not the clock-ticking etc. (see above). I've accepted the chance that I would never marry because I couldn't have children. In my mind ALL men want is children, or every opportunity to make children, right?

I have a wonderful job, I'm not married, and I'm pretty much free to do as I wish (yeah, I know what you're thinking: a married woman's worse nightmare). I should be on top of the world. Several of my friends that are still married are pregnant and the ones that aren't pregnant are getting divorced. So I'm thinking, "Do they really have it better than me?" HELLO!! I begin looking at myself in the mirror each day and thanking God for sparing my life.

Now I have gotten where I stay tired all the time and there is no reason for it. My hair is shedding; my weight is up and down. (Not thunder thighs again.) There is NO reason to go to the ob-gyn on this one, so I've got to find a family doctor. All I can think is, here I go again.

Well, I make an appointment with a doctors group and my appointment is with a woman. All I could think is "WOW!" a doctor that's female (not to be confused with a female doctor). This won't be embarrassing at all.

I began telling her all of my symptoms and she asks about my health history. When I started telling her everything she was blown away (thank goodness Cross pens makes refills; hell I can't even write without a prescription inference). Then she asks me when my last pap smear was. I looked at her and said, "Not since my post-op checkup years ago, why?" She advises me that I should have a smear at least every two years because I could get vaginal cancer. Now wouldn't that be just great to have to lose the play, after they have already taken the pen? Then she noticed a rash under my skin on the right side of my neck and face. I thought that was from the sun or blood blisters from something. She tells me to go to the lab for some blood test. As if; great, the vampire thing again.

I go to the lab, which is right around the corner, and the

lab technician starts getting the needles and tubes ready for the blood draw. When she comes to me with the needle, I say, "My veins are wiped out due to all the surgery, so they will run and hide, but if you put your thumb on one and push down you can get as much blood as you want." Did she listen? NO! So she stuck me once, twice and finally, on the third stick, she did as I told her and guess what? She actually got the tubes filled with blood. I said, "Told you." Now what is so hard about "hearing" what a patient says? Nothing! Again, here is where we know our bodies.

I go home, wait on her to call me with my results from the vampire. Several days later I still haven't heard. I am still exhausted, so I call her. When she returns my call, she tells me I need to come back in to talk. Whenever I have heard this kind of news, it's never been good. So my emotions start to rise again.

I make the appointment, the day comes and my heart is racing, my emotions are crazy, and my mind is wandering everywhere. They call me back to the exam room and my doctor comes in and says, "Your blood pressure is a little high today." Go figure, I'm scared to death. All I can think is, "Get To The Point!" I'm thinking I'm just tired, give me a vitamin, and let me go home. She tells me I have your test results and there are some concerns. Okay, just tell me. I can handle it! She tells me that the results are: Lupus, fibromyalgia, anemia, and an under-active thyroid. I've been hit in the head with the dumb brick, what in the crap is all of this?

I take a deep breath, and say, "So what do we do?" She says, "We treat the symptoms, the thyroid can be controlled with synthroid." Treat the symptoms? Well let's see, how? I don't even know what half of this stuff means. I get more prescriptions, and here I thought my body was finished being probed and being used as guinea pig, silly me.

In my mind I know I can handle this and I will not let it beat me. I have been through way too much to stop fighting now.

Now I'm wondering what to do next and, a bit of good news, I get promoted at work, love my new job and throw myself into it. I'm still not satisfied with my life; you know, the husband thing. See I'm about 31 years old now, I don't want people to think, you know. Not that anything is wrong with it; it's just not me. You are probably wondering what all of this has to do with knowing your body. Stay with me and you will understand.

Now understand, in my job I have seen it all: unruly children (makes me glad not to have kids), alcoholics, sexually abused adults and children, domestics (husband/wife, boyfriend/girlfriend fights), death, fire, sexual predators and much more. Oh, my job, sorry, forgot to tell you, I'm a dispatcher for 911. I have also helped officers by searching females for drugs on the scene of meth labs and other drug searches. I have been in some of the most awful homes, sitting and waiting for the Department of Children's Services to come and pick up children because of abuse, drugs or worse. See, now I can help people and think so much about what else can happen to me. So I put my energy into trying to help others. I see that life is not so great for a lot of other people in the world.

I have a wonderful job (did I mention that already); my health is not tearing me down to the point of screaming and thinking about it all the time. I have met a nice man and we begin dating. (See, there is hope for me yet!) We actually have a lot in common; he is a police officer for the same county, and my best friend is also his partner. We date for a while, before I tell him that I'm not able to have children. He has two children by his first marriage, a boy and a girl. I finally get to meet his children and I fall head over heels for both of them. They were so sweet the first time I met them, even though they were his children by another woman. I only have love for them both. After dating for a while he asked me to marry him. As bad as I wanted to get married and have a family, I was scared to death. He kept telling me it didn't matter that I couldn't have children, he had two and that's all he wanted (and it really wasn't the child support thing, I promise) plus, he was so sweet about it all. I finally told him yes and we are married on May 25, 1996 (of course I remember and yes, I know you know I'm divorced because I mentioned it earlier). Now I'm a married woman, if I get the picket fence, well two out of three ain't bad.

It was a beautiful wedding. We were married at my aunt's house, which faced a lake with lots of flowers she had growing in her yard. We were surrounded with family and friends and held the reception outside as well. It was a beautiful day. I had my family and friends and a man that loves me, even though I'm half a woman on the inside. That night on our honeymoon, I never felt so beautiful and felt like a real woman again. My life seemed like it was back on track again. He knew everything about me and still loved me.

I have begun to really love married life, my little family (even though it is only part-time), and my job. My life is really looking up. I love being a mother, even though I'm only a stepmother. The kids loved being with us, even though his son didn't get to be with us as much as his daughter because he was born with a very rare disease that caused his immune system to be very low. Since he can't fight off anything and also has a feeding tube, he has to be hooked up to a feeding pump with special vitamins and has special needs in other aspects of his life. The time with him is always special. I have learned a lot from him at this point; he is ALWAYS happy, ALWAYS, and takes what life throws at him, regardless. That is one thing he taught me, that someone, somewhere, has to deal with more than I had to.

I have been married a little over a year. I'm in the shower, checking my breasts for any abnormalities because of all the estrogen I have to take. To all of you who are still with me, you should take notice of any changes in your body even if you think it's small. My husband (if I am remembering right), okay, okay, I know he is my husband, was sitting on the end of our bed putting his socks on for work, and he heard me scream. While I was checking my right breast, blood and some thick green stuff came out of my areola. (NIPPLE) he came running in the bathroom and said, "What in the world is wrong with you?" I opened the shower curtain, standing there in disbelief, with big mule tears rolling down my face. He grabbed my robe, put me in the car, and to the emergency room we go. I didn't know what to think at this point, but he kept reassuring me everything would be okay.

We arrive at the hospital and after filling out a small book of paperwork, the nurse and doctor come into the room. They start by asking all these questions, like, "Have you been hit in the chest?" Now understand I would know if I had been hit in the chest just as if a man would know if he had been hit in the balls (sorry, not a medical term, I know). If they asked me that once, they asked me ten times. What part of NO did they not understand? So they began pushing on my nipple and stuff was just rolling out. The doctor tells me I need to see a surgeon.

DUH! My husband even knew that before they checked me, and he is a cop not a doctor.

The hospital calls in a general surgeon; he tells me I have an infected milk duct, and he will have to remove it. (The milk duct, not the tit.) I'm okay with that, so we prepare for surgery. Thinking they will come and get me, take me to the operating room and put me to sleep, right? WRONG!

The nurse starts preparing my breast and nipple with Betadine and drapes a cloth over my chest and face. My husband at this point is outside pacing the hallway and all I can think about at this point is, I want my mom!

Now it's time for the surgeon to come in and I'm wondering how much of this am I going to feel? Any other surgery I've had I've been asleep and felt nothing until I woke up. You are thinking, she is older and wiser, right? I may be older, but stupid when it comes to surgery to the breast. The doctor tells me to take a deep breath and that I will feel a big sting. What the crap is he saying? Has he ever had surgery on his nipple? I don't think so! He started putting needles with numbing medication right to the nipple. Ouch! Understand, a woman's milk duct is small; when he removed mine it looked like a shrimp. YUM! Just kidding. I get my stitches, ice pack and go home. I was told the "shrimp" would be sent off to the pathology department and to come back to get my stitches removed in seven to ten days.

The pathology report comes back as just what it was, an infected milk duct. My stitches are removed and I feel like another weight has been lifted off my chest (no pun intended). Several months go by and the same thing happens again. I know this is not normal so I make an appointment with a plastic surgeon. I take my doctor's notes from the first surgery to him. Now brace yourself for this one. My husband and I are sitting in his office after the examination waiting on the doctor to come and talk to us.

The doctor walks in the door. My heart is racing. He sits down behind his desk and leans back in his big chair, and says, "yes, it is another infected milk duct. We will remove it, and it is most likely caused by your husband's saliva (spit.)" I looked at him like he had lost his mind. My husband came unglued. At the same time we both said, "If this is true just about every woman that has had sex would be losing milk ducts, and (oh, btw) his spit didn't hurt his first wife (yeah, I know, a little too much info)." We got up and left his office faster than rabbits! Get it? I told my husband that doctor is like a pop tart, "jelly filled brain!" We went home and made two appointments with two other doctors to get a second and third opinion.

Had you been told this by a renowned plastic surgeon, would you want other opinions? Renowned or not, I did!!!!

So now I have two appointments for my breast. Scared to death, my husband is upset hoping it's not his fault because of what the first surgeon said. That would upset any man that loved his woman. We made the two appointments just several hours apart, to ease both our minds. Two doctors in one day, but I felt it is very necessary to be 100 percent sure of what the outcome would be. If they gave us different diagnoses then we decided to see another doctor (listen to your gut feeling as well as your body).

We are sitting with doctor #2 (remember #1 is the spit doctor), I'm in the exam room talking to the doctor and he's laughing about the spit theory. Doctor #2 sends me for a mammogram, ultrasound and a test where the radiologist stuck needles with special wires right into the nipple, and then with the wires and needle still attached I get another mammary gram (for those who have never had one, this is an x-ray that smashes your tit to a flat pancake). I know a man had everything to do with inventing this test, including the needle thing 'cause a woman would have better sense. Someday a woman MUST invent a penis gram and yes, with the needle, just like the one we have each year. Don't ya think??

All test are complete, I'm thinking it'll be days before we get results, but not true. The doctor comes in and goes over everything with us right then. He says, "You need a mastectomy, it does not look good." (I'm thinking, "you need to be castrated, I bet yours doesn't look good, sorta tit-for-that.) We decide to go to doctor #3 at this point.

Doctor #3, and you will not believe this, was a woman! I felt like Godwas finally helping me out here. I gave her all the x-rays from doctors #1 and #2. She was very compassionate with everything I had gone through. My husband was sitting in the waiting room and at this point he'd had all he could take with doctors. She sat and talked with me like I was the only patient she had in her office. I appreciated the time she was taking in explaining options to me. I looked at her with tears (oh yeah, the mule ones) and asked her, "If this was happening to you or your daughter, what would you do?" She answered, "I would have the complete mastectomy." I took a deep breath and she says, "Take a few minutes. I will get your husband." My tears are rolling like a waterfall (they were not like the ones in Hawaii). She did tell me that the problem with my right breast is NOT caused from my husband's spit and he was happy to hear this. I cry for a good half hour, then pull myself together after reassurance from my husband that my health is more important than a titty.

Surgery is scheduled for September 11, 2001 at 5:00 a.m. We arrived at the hospital and the nurses begin prepping me. I just thought I was scared when I had my ob-gyn surgeries, now I'm horrified about this surgery because the other surgeries were not on the outside where it was going to be noticeable (call it vanity if you wish). I'd already lost so much womanhood; now my breast is being cut off (no, I don't want to hear from some man, he can only pay attention to one breast at a time and more than a mouthful is a waste—don't try that one with me). I know what you women are thinking: "Why didn't you elect to do reconstruction right after the surgery?" My doctor told me if I allow the mastectomy to heal, then elect for reconstruction, I'd have a better chance of the reconstruction taking the first time. I've been prepped and am only waiting to go down to the operating room. My mom, husband and stepfather, (yes, mom remarried to a wonderful, caring man) are at the end of my bed telling me everything will be fine. My dad and brother have not made it to the hospital at this time, but are on their way. (I'm hoping to see them both before they take me down, just in case "something" happens.)

As the nurse calls over the intercom to tell us they will be right up to take me down to surgery, I look up and my dad and brother are walking in, I know my sigh of relief was obvious. I tell them all how much I love them and don't worry. Yeah, like they weren't already scared and worried. The team comes to get me and I look at my family, we're all crying. At that moment I just told them all to pray!

Surgery is over (it took several hours) and the team brings me back to the room where my family was waiting. I've awaken though still dazed from the drug and I ask what movie are they watching on television? When I was told that the World Trade Center's Twin Towers had been attacked by terrorists, my breast did not seem so important anymore. If we all look around when bad things happens to us, someone has always had something worse happen to them. Usually, it makes me think my problems are pretty small (At least the right side of my chest).

Don't misunderstand, the pain is tremendous and I've already called for a pain shot. When the nurse brings the shot, she wants to look at my bandage (I've not seen it yet), and she wants to empty my drainage tube (I didn't know I had one). Now this is the first time I ever felt like I was going to be sick. It's disgusting (the reddish fluid in the drainage tube bulb is so gross). The fluid has a distinctive smell (not like roses) more like a skunk with diarrhea (not that I've been around a lot of them—skunks, I mean).

It's around 7:00 p.m. and they come in to tell my family it's time for everyone to leave, including my husband. I had a screaming, crying fit. I wasn't about to stay alone in that hospital. Finally to settle me down, they allowed my husband to stay with me through the night. I called for pain shots every four hours but they never really eased the pain. Under my arm, around my back, I just hurt all over. Morning finally comes and all I want to do is go home to sleep in my own bed. When my doctor comes in I ask, "Can I go?" She advises me that just as soon as I learn to empty the drainage tube and am taught my exercises, I can. As disgusting as it is, I emptied the bulb and learned to walk my arm (yes, I realize I said walk an arm) up and down the wall. Even though it hurts like hell, I try to hide it 'cause all I want to do is leave this hellhole.

Finally, I have my release papers, a pain shot, four pillows and I'm on my way home. It's a 60-mile trip to get home, and I'm so glad I've got pillows and extra glad to be going home. The ride home is not the easiest ride in the world (a pothole may be a pothole, but have a boob taken off and a pothole...

well, just don't believe all those tire commercials about smooth rides). Finally we get home, my husband helps me in the door (so my dogs won't jump on me) and I plop down in the recliner, where I stay for the next seven days.

My husband is pretty swell about the whole thing. On the other hand, it's me having problems coping with it all, from the drainage tubes to taking a shower and getting dressed. I had a terrible outlook on pretty much everything. I know I'm the only person in the world having to go through all of this. Boy, am I crazy or what? But that's how I felt, crazy and alone!

The more my husband and family tried to help me, it seemed, the more resentment I showed toward them. Even when the American Cancer Society comes to my house to offer me support (no pun intended), a prosthesis and bra, I'm even rude to them. I knew in my heart this wasn't me, but it seemed like I had no control over my emotions and my MOUTH! (I was having diarrhea of the mouth at this point and had also forgotten most of the King's English) Anything that anyone tried to do for me was never good enough (does the word B-I-O-T-C-H come to mind?). It was the "for me" that got to me, I believe.

My mom was driving 50 miles one way to come and help me while my husband was at work. I treated her so awful! To this day, I feel awful because of the way I talked to her. She understood that it wasn't "me", it was anger and, by God, I believed I had earned it. She kept coming everyday, just like clockwork! (That's a mother's love.) When my husband got home from work it was shift-time, when mom leaves and husband begins. He was great, too, but in my heart and mind, I wanted my mother.

My mom and my husband were sooooo great! It was me that was so very, very awful! When it was time for my tubing to be stripped and the bulb to be emptied, neither one of them would complain about having to do this, even though it stunk to high heaven (refer back to the skunk theory). As long as the drainage was 50cc a day, the doctor would not remove the drainage tube. Finally, the drainage subsided to below the 50cc mark for two days and I called my doctor. She advised me to come in and it would be removed. (I still haven't looked at my chest since the mastectomy). I have this tight bandage around my chest and whenever my mom or my husband would remove it, I would just close my eyes. This is the day I'll have to look and I'm really, really, really, (three reallys means FOR REAL) not ready for this.

The nurse comes in the room and the first thing she says is, "How are you doing?" I bust out crying! "Where does it hurt?" she asks. All I can say is, "My heart!"(No, I'm not having a heart attack). I'm lying down on the exam table and she removes the bandage, (thank goodness I was lying down, or I would have probably fainted). I raise my head to look at my chest to see that I have a large tube, attached by stitches, to my chest. My chest has a long scar from the center of my chest to my underarm. No nipple and I'm as flat as the top of a table (not a pancake, 'cause a pancake actually has a little puff to it). I'm in such shock I can't even cry.

When the doctor comes in, she says, "This looks great.. What the hell kinda meds is she on???!!!! She removes the stitches holding the tube in place and tells me to take a deep breath so she can pull the tube out. When the tube is removed, I'm in a daze (damn, I now know what a field line to a septic tank must feel like) because it took a whole lot of tubing to carry that shit out of my body. She tells me that it was all the way around to my shoulder bone. Why, I ask? Fluid can build up around the complete side and under the arm and this helps to reduce the chance for infection. The stitches across my chest area aren't ready to be removed. As if that doesn't look bad enough, now I've got to keep looking at where my breast was supposed to be, with stitches, scabs, and the bruising. She advises me that if any puffiness shows up around the incision to call her immediately because this means fluid is building up and it will have to be drained off (probably another large needle, no doubt).

Mom is now driving me home; I'm sitting in the car saying absolutely nothing, staring out the window, not even thinking about anything, just back in that dazed state. No anger, no feelings whatsoever.

Mom keeps asking, "Are you okay? "Yes, Momma," I reply, not in a hateful voice, in a soft, confused one. She calls the doctor when we got to my house, worried about my mental state at this point. I've gone from being MS BIOTCH to not saying anything (she has been through so much with me, but has never seen me speechless). When the doctor calls her back, she reassures her that all the emotions I'm showing are pretty much normal. She tells my mom that I will go through several stages: fear, anger, grieving, possibly after all these I'll be emotionally drained (ya think!!!!). That's when you sleep a lot (I call that depressed). My mom knows me better than anyone. She's not only my mom, she's my best friend (please no psychological babble on the mom/best friend thing, I'm not a child anymore, so we can actually be friends). My husband at this point doesn't know what to do with my emotional roller coaster. He tries to be there for me but I just want to be left alone.

If any of you have a bathtub mirror facing the tub, BIG MISTAKE! Let me explain...as long as the drainage tube was in, I had to take a shower, because you can't sit in the tub. My shower is separate from my bathtub, so no mirror. I was ready to sit in a long hot bath, even though I couldn't lie down in the water and that's exactly what I did. When I'm ready to stand up with the help of my husband, there's the big mirror. I have to see what I really look like because of that damned mirror. If my husband hadn't been helping me, I know I would have fallen. It's the most god ugly thing I've ever seen. Why would he want to stay with me? I'm deformed! I want to crawl in a hole and stay there. Hibernation would be a good thing since I've been a grizzly bear to everyone I've come in contact with! ("She-Devil.") I wonder if I will ever get back to the happy, go-lucky person I was before all of this. I am wishing at this point that I knew someone that had gone through this misery or some thing to read besides medical terminology. Not so lucky!!

Now you know WHY I'm trying (note, trying) to be a writer! Since I've been to hell and back, hopefully I can explain the trip, you know, kinda like a tour guide at the morgue (you don't really want to be there, but somebody has to do it) and maybe, just maybe, this might help someone else someday!

I'm still mad at the world! When I take my bath I turn facing the wall until I get dried off and put my robe on immediately. I have a walk-in closet so I get dressed in it. I never make love to my husband anymore, unless I have a tee shirt on and it stays on. I've lost weight, down to about 98 pounds. I'm really a mess! My best friend never calls anymore because she can't handle seeing me hurt (what kind of crap is she trying to pull?) and all I can think is, the time I need her most, why can't she be there? I lie in bed at night while my husband is working and cry uncontrollably. I have family members telling me, "There is NO reason to have reconstruction, you look great." Yeah, right! Of course, family isn't going to give you a complex. My brother was all for the reconstruction. He tells me that I'm a beautiful woman and if that's what I want there should be NO question. Just go for it! So that is exactly what I decided to do!

Now I've got a decision to make about the reconstruction surgery. The doctor that did the mastectomy has a partner that is a plastic surgeon. A little luck, finally! I trust her judgment. I'm still dealing with the lupus and all the other things, and now I've got this to think about, so I make the appointment with the plastic surgeon. I hate the thought of being put to sleep again, but I hate the way I look even more.

I have gotten several brochures from the doctor to read about reconstruction surgeries. There are two options that I have to consider.

One is called a TRAM FLAP. (Wondering what this means?) I can explain…A Tram Flap (in my words) begins with the doctor cutting your abdomen (where a tummy tuck would be) taking the muscle, tissue and blood veins and twisting them from the left side up to the right side of the chest. (OUCH!) When this procedure is done I only have one chance of it working. If the blood supply dies, then the surgery is null and void and I will have to wait six months before anything else can be thought about.

I will have drainage tubes (yes, field line analogy time again) not only in my chest area, but also in my abdomen area and I know how gross those are! My brother is a big man, but he did the sweetest thing, since I would only have one chance with this type of reconstruction, he offered me his tissue and muscle (yes, he has plenty to spare). My doctor told me that most of the time tissue from a sibling is NOT a match, and it's very hard to take tissue for this type of surgery from a non-relative and keep the tissue alive.

The second option is a tissue expander and then an implant. This sounds like it would be easier on my body and me. This procedure will take a lot longer to see results, though. Now a tissue expander is "implant like." The doctor will put this in, put in saline (water) and fill the expander over several visits to stretch my tissue so an implant will fit under my skin. Sounds simple, right? That's what I'm thinking too, simple! Like I said earlier, this procedure may take a little longer, but the Tram Flap is just too risky. (My opinion only.)

I guess you have figured out that I chose the tissue expander/implant. Now I wonder how they will make my left even with my right. I'm in the doctor's office where there are several other ladies in the waiting room. I'm wondering if any of them are going through breast reconstruction. I'm holding my shoulders forward (yes, the stooped look) and my head down so no one will NOTICE I have a deformity. I've got on a big sweatshirt and jeans so you can't SEE why I'm there. The nurse comes out to the waiting room telling me to come on back. She takes me to the exam room and great, there are mirrors all over one wall. I freeze! I ask, "Why are there so many mirrors?" She replies, "It's so the doctor can show you what he will be doing." In the back of my mind all I could think of is, well, he can look but I'm not. My mom is with me (my husband had to work) and she says, "It's okay, I'm right here." I started to cry (you would think by now I'd taken out stock in Kleenex). It seems like she is always so strong and there for me regardless of what happens. (I really do realize my mom is my best friend.) The nurse gives me a robe to put on, not paper, but a nice blue and white stripped one with a belt to wrap around my waist. I'm thinking this is pretty cool since I had paper gowns at the ob-gyn. I'm now sitting on the end of the table, and in walks the man who will change my life. (In all reality, I am the one who changed my life; he was my angel who made that happen.) He shakes my hand, introduces himself and I remember his hands being so soft. This is where my life begins again.

He's wearing a crisp white coat with dark blue pants and is toting a box with a lid on it. He tells me to stand up and open my robe. He just looks and tells me I can belt the robe back and have a seat. He opens the box and there are several different sizes of implants, none the size of my petite left breast. (They don't make them that small.). He tells me about a law, which was passed several years ago, which states that all insurance companies HAVE to pay to fix the opposite breast to match the mastectomy. I had no idea of this law. He hands me a packet of papers to read and shows me the tissue expander and the implant he would recommend to be portioned with my body. They both are kind of shaped like a teardrop. He then explains that when I had the breast removed they also removed the muscle, so a pocket will have to be built up to hold the implant in place. My fear and sadness have left, now I've gotten excited that maybe my breast-less area can be fixed. I asked, "What about the nipple?" He tells me that will be way down the road and not to worry about that right now. It will take several months to fill the expander once it's put in and then I will have to be larger on that side for at least a month (once its full) to stretch the tissue. I say lets get started! I get dressed and I'm put in a room with his nurse to schedule surgery.

Mom and I go to the car, start the drive home and I can't stop talking about everything. I call my husband to tell him and he says, "You sound so good, are you okay?" why YES I am, he can fix me a breast!

Mom is driving because I'm still not allowed to drive yet.

Why? Because I can't wear a seatbelt and get this, my surgeon has given me a doctor's note so if we get stopped or involved in a wreck they won't write me a ticket for not wearing a seatbelt. I never realized there is so much to all of this, bet you didn't either. I have good doctors; they are the ones that think of everything.

We get home; I have a message to come to the sheriff's office for our yearly pictures. Yeah, right! I'm short, so you know I'll be in the front row, no way am I going to have my picture made for any calendar. I call my boss, who is also a great friend, who tells me no one will be able to tell, get dressed and be there the next day. I've not been back to work since the mastectomy (I took a leave of absence) and all I can think is that everyone is going to stare. Silly, I know! I'm a supervisor over the dispatchers and a lot of them had been to the house to see me, but none of the officers, who are all males, so I guess I can see why they stayed away, I mean geeeezzzz what would we talk about? But I will have to face them too. I'm not so sure about this. I tell my boss I'll think about it. He must have told several of the employees because my phone started ringing and being who I am, I give in and go. Guess what? It wasn't so bad after all, matter of fact, I even smiled!!!

The day for the expander surgery has finally arrived. I get up at 4:00 a.m. and I'm so nervous, I get sick to my stomach. My mind is running wild. I'm sure you can relate to most of it. I fill out all the paperwork, and then the nurse calls me back to the prep room. (What are they going to prep, there's nothing there!) My doctor comes into the prep room where I've already had the IV put in my arm and tells me he has to mark where he will be working. (He used a purple magic marker, Scripto I think, maybe Marks-A-Lot and I would have preferred pink.) I stand up straight (been awhile since I did this) and he marks where he'll be cutting the center of my chest. It's time to go into the operating room and while I'm scared to death, I'm also excited that the reconstruction is finally beginning. I get on the table and the nurse starts putting on the heart monitors and a blood pressure cuff. She tells me not to ever have my blood pressure taken on the side of the mastectomy and while this is the first time I've heard this it's good to know, because it can cause serious problems that I was not aware of. For one, you won't get a true reading on you blood pressure, and it can cause a blood clot and numbness. So anyone going through this beware! They tell me to count backwards from 100. I may have gotten to 98. (Sweet Dreams.)

Eventually, they call my family and tell them I'm in recovery and they can see me in an hour. I'm thinking, it has only been about 30 minutes and I hear my mom coming through the recovery room doors. The nurse tells her she can't be back here, but my mom tells her, "That's my daughter and it's been 2 ½ hours and I want to know why we haven't been called." My blood pressure had dropped very low and the nurses were working to get it back up. Needless to say, mom got to stay with me in recovery.

I'm in a bunch of pain (a bunch of pain is more than a little, but not more than one can endure) and my chest feels like I imagine an overfilled water balloon might feel. It's throbbing and burning like fire (okay, a water balloon might not feel like fire, but you get my meaning). The nurses can't give me a lot of pain meds until my blood pressure gets up. So an ice bag becomes my friend. Have you ever heard the phrase, "It's colder than a witch's titty in a tin bra?" Well, I'm feeling like a witch—with a B, so maybe this is where that phrase comes from.

I guess it froze my new titty (welcome to my world, new titty) because my blood pressure finally comes up to normal and although I'm enduring the pain the nurse gives me a shot. How do you spell RELIEF???? I spell it Demerol, and oh what a relief it is.

Later that night I can go home. Insurance companies are really hard on patients and what they think is appropriate recovery time from surgery. Ready for this, I bet you a doughnut to a dollar, it was a man who figured out that one breast removal = one day in the hospital. Hell, he probably thought, she's got another one anyway. Most of you already know this. We pay high premiums and they tell us what to do or they won't pay. IN MY OPINION I THINK THEY NEED TO SIT DOWN AND SHUT UP. But I digress and that's a whole different story...

Now I get to go home, ice packs, antibiotics, pain meds and a pillow. I thought the pain was bad before, lord have mercy, am I wrong. This is horrible. I can't even think of an example to let you all know how bad it hurts. I keep a daily journal, well, maybe not so daily, but pretty close and the words I used to describe the pain, well, even with what you've already read me use, I can't use these words now and I even get disturbed with myself when I read from back then. It was just awful, take my word for it. I think, how in the world am I going to be ready for the doctor to put more solution into this expander in seven to ten days? I have gotten zero sleep in two days and I finally just pass out because I'm so tired. The pain wakes me up in about two hours; I take the pain meds and sit in the recliner to sleep. When four or five days pass, so did the pain. Now it's time to make my next appointment.

I go back to the doctor in about eight days. He and his

nurse come in with a bag of saline water and a butterfly needle. (A butterfly needle is a small needle with green like wings.) He takes a magnet and swings it over my hump in my chest. I have no idea what this "magnet swinging" thing is all about but I did think of a refrigerator. Finally the magnet attaches to my skin (I kid you not), he tells me this is where the wire mesh is for the fill up. "Fill up." Now I've gone from feeling like a refrigerator, to flunking a metal detector in an airport, to "filling up" like you'd gas up your car in a matter of five minutes. This allows him to hit the spot on the first try. The butterfly needle is inserted into my expander (which looks like a bald head, that's my dig to guys, not babies) and the fill up begins. He tells me to say STOP when I can't take the pressure any more. He had put in approximately 75cc and I scream, "STOP!" He takes the needle out and puts a band-aid on the small hole. His nurse, one of the sweetest people I've ever met, asks, "Are you okay?" I reply, "I think so. I was expecting it to be a lot worse." She gives me a prescription for pain meds and tells me "you will need these later on tonight." Mom drives me home and my husband goes to the pharmacy. Sure enough, I was glad to have the meds later that night. The pain showed up just like she said. My chest hurt, my back, even under my arm. I'm thinking how many more fill ups can I stand.

My lupus decides to flare up so now I've got muscle spasms and joint pain along with titty, the new one, pain. My family doctor, who treats the lupus, calls in a muscle relaxer and a steroid. I get relief from all of it and sleep.

My husband takes a second job as a police chief to keep me from worrying about work and bills. He wants me to only concentrate on getting better. So he is working two jobs, because I'm facing at least two more surgeries.

I can't say I know many men that would do this for their significant other, do you?

I return to the doctor several times for more fill ups (when you stop and think about the terminology "fill ups" its really hard not to laugh, wouldn't you agree?) and the same pain and misery. We've all heard the old saying, "No pain, no gain." For the pain I'm going through, I pray it is worth it. Finally my expander is full; it's so large compared to the other side. I really look funny with one baldheaded titty, the size of a large cantaloupe and the other side the size of a fluffy homemade roll. Now I have to wait for the skin (yeah, the skin above all those fill ups) to get elasticity. It will take up to three months or longer. At this point I hope time flies!

Time does not fly, we all know this, but I get through not three months but four. I return to the doctor, he tells me I'm ready for the expander to be removed and the implant to be put in, which is absolutely wonderful news. Maybe now I will not be so uneven and self-conscious. Then I can get over this surgery and hopefully go back to work. I had someone come up to me in a store and ask, "Did you have your breast amputated?" I replied, "I guess you could say that." Some people do NOT have a clue!!!! I can laugh about that now.

Surgery is scheduled!!! I'm finally at the stage where I can be normal looking in my clothes. I will look okay in a bathing suit (vanity, I know). I just won't have a nipple on that side (oh well, no more wet t-shirt contest for me). I go to the outpatient surgery center and wait for the nurse to call my name. I'm sitting in the waiting room, looking at a magazine, but not really seeing it, waiting and waiting. Finally the nurse comes out and calls me back to the pre-op room. I've been through this so many times, but I'm still anxious at this point. All the preparations and pain of the past few months are fixing (no pun intended) to be a BIG payoff, at least to me. Hopefully, no more hiding in the closet to get dressed and no more avoiding mirrors.

My angel of hope walks in with his magic marker! (Yep, the same color!!) I'm sure a lot of you have watched "The Swan" or "Extreme Makeover," and have seen how they mark what they are going to fix, that's how I'm marked. I put the beautiful (now that was a pun) blue "shower cap" on and in the operating room we go. This is it! I can't wait to wake up from surgery and see my results.

I'm in recovery and my husband and mom are trying to talk to me so I'll wake up. The nurses will not release you until you get up and pee. I guess to make sure all the plumbing is working. I finally wake up and all I want is to see my new breast. My doctor has put another one of those tight wraps around my chest and I can't see a thing, but I can feel the pain. Oh boy, does it hurt. The wrap feels like it's cutting off my air supply. No pain, no gain, right?

I'm released to go home, the nurse gives me a big ole pain shot and I try to sleep on the way. My husband is worried because I keep complaining about the wrap being too tight. He calls the doctor (aren't cell phones just wonderful at times) and he tells him it can come off the next day. Needless to say, I don't know if I'll make it to the next day. It is really hurting. We get home, again I camp out in the recliner, and it's easier to get up and down. I feel like I'm starting over. I know in my heart this isn't starting over, it's a new beginning.

I finally get to take off the wrap. I DO NOT do this in front of a mirror. I have to work up my nerve to look. I was brave in the recovery room, but now I feel like a chicken. My husband is so kind and reassuring, he's telling me how good my breast reconstruction looks. He helps me get the nerve to look at myself. It takes me several hours, but I go to the mirror, unbutton my pajama top, take a deep breath and look. Besides looking like a bald head, (no nipple, remember?) my normal breast and it match up pretty great. I feel my shoulders straighten up instead of being slumped over a bit. I kinda even get a smile on my face. I ask my husband to get my bathing suit top (when all else fails, vanity—okay); I want to see if I look normal in it. (Whatever "normal" is.) I put it on, I can see the mastectomy scar under my arm a little, but other than that, it looks just like a boob. I put my pajama top back on and go back to my recliner with a sigh of relief. It worked better than I thought!

I feel great about myself for the next year or so. I'm thinking I'm on top of the world. I go back to work; heck, I even get a second job with one of my best friends in her café. I don't feel like I have to hide anymore. Oh, I know what's underneath my clothes isn't perfect, but the way I feel about myself is, well, not too shabby.

I have an appointment with my family doctor who's located in another town some fours hours away, in a couple of weeks. She will be so surprised! Of course she knows about the surgery, but she hasn't seen the results of it yet. My husband and I have a good friend and his girlfriend over for dinner and a movie. I feel like my life is finally on track and back to normal (I know, that word again, look, just put "_" around it yourself). I feel good around family and friends again. I feel like I can be the wife my husband expected when we were married. He's been so great and understanding. So, they come over for dinner (have you ever had a feeling in your stomach, that makes you feel like your going to throw up and you can't put your finger on it?) we eat and start watching a movie. The feeling in my stomach just isn't going away, but why? They are all acting so strange, except for her boyfriend (now you know who the "they" are). Are you all still with me? This is where, once again, I learned to follow my gut feeling.

At this point I feel like my life is meaningful and happy again. Mom and I go to my doctor's appointment (out of town, but, I've set a voice-activated tape recorder on my phone, just to see if my gut feeling is real or stupid. All the way to my doctor I keep telling mom I know I'm just being stupid. He would never cheat on me. NEVER! We have been through so much together. If he was going to destroy our marriage by cheating, he would have done it when I was having my breast cut off. Right?

She just keeps assuring me not to be so negative in my thinking. It's just something that does not feel kosher (more like a sour dill pickle). I decide to enjoy our four-hour trip and worry when there's something to worry about.

We are at our destination, check into the hotel room, and get ready to go out for supper. I call home and tell him we made it okay and he is just as sweet as pie. Maybe I'm stupid?? Maybe not?? I'll know in about 36 hours. Mom and I go out to eat and looking around. I have an early doctor's appointment so we return to the hotel and go to bed. I get up and go to my doctor and go through a lot of blood tests. We talk about my surgery; she looks at my reconstruction and tells me he did beautiful work. I don't have to deal with one of my insecurities (my breast), at least that's off my list. My lab results, well, I'll have to wait until they come back from pathology. As for my husband, I'll know if I'm being stupid in about seven hours. We get on the road home and the closer I get to home, the more butterflies I get in my stomach (thank God these butterflies didn't have needles attached to them, because I would have certainly bled out if they did). I'll never forget that feeling, sick and scared. I'm hoping the man I love so much, hasn't done anything to make me act like the "Ultimate She-Devil!" but, the closer we get to my house, the sicker I feel. I actually don't have any reason to feel this way at this time. Just my gut feeling! WHEN YOU HAVE A GUT FEELING, FOLLOW IT!

We finally get home and pull in my driveway; my heart feels like it is going to jump out of my chest (Yeah, yeah, I know what you're thinking, hope the scars hold....right?) I go into the house and let the dogs out and mom goes outside in the backyard to sit on the swing. I go to my bedroom and pull the tape recorder out from under the bed. I rewind it (not even all the way) and push play.... what did I hear? My husband on the phone with a woman talking about sex and what they are going to do once he moves out.

I knew her voice; she is the so-called friend that sat at my kitchen table a few weeks before eating my food. I began to cry. (Yes, MULE TEARS) I'm really not sure at this time if I am crying because it hurt so badly or if I was just that damn angry. When we got married there was only ONE thing I asked of him, if you feel the urge to cheat, just tell me. If you do cheat, you will get DIVORCE papers. He swore that he had been hurt in the same manner and would never do this to me. His first wife cheated on him with a good friend of his.

Back to the story of my life! After hearing such sick stuff, I rewind the tape all the way. I go out and sit on the swing; by this time my mom had called my dad. I ask both of them to go inside the house while I listen to my husband and his trollop talk. I'm sitting in the swing, I really can't tell you how long, staring at the buffalo and the pond. I still have not listened to the entire tape. Finally I turned the tape on and started listening. It had the most hurtful things on it. She tells him that she will have to get a new television so her kids will have something to do while they are having sex. What kind of mother is that? Then I hear him tell her to hold on, that I'm beeping in on the other line, he answers like he is asleep, tells me he loves me and hangs up, when he returns on the line with her she starts laughing. She is laughing because he tells her, oh that was her (ME), and she says what the hell did she want? Wait a minute, I call my husband at my house and she asks what I wanted. What is that? I think I rewind that part several times.

I keep listening, and the tape conversation goes on for over four hours. All of it makes me want to throw up on him.

He is at work, I call his cell phone, and I act like nothing is wrong. (Talk about hard to do.) I tell him he needs to come home right now! I ask him what part of the county he is in; he's in the area where SHE lives. He tells me he's on his way, what's wrong? I tell him think about it on the way home and see if you can figure it out.

I wipe the tears from my face, go into the house, my parents sitting at the kitchen table and I tell them he is on his way home, please just be here for me. I'll take care of the rest. I don't want to pull them into my problem. My parents are always there for my brother and me. This I had to do on my own.

It seems like an hour since I called him to tell him to come home (only 10 minutes), so I call him again. He tells me he is on his way. I tell him he has about five minutes and if he isn't here everything he owns (clothes) will be on fire in the driveway. He is still acting like he has no clue (to me) what is wrong. Being a deputy you would think he would have been a little smarter, since I work at the sheriff's office too. See, that is an advantage, I can check his radio traffic anytime. How hard is it to notice a green and white patrol car sitting somewhere, like her driveway?

He comes in the front door, I think I'm really mad now, and asked, "Can I talk to you in the bedroom?" "Sure, you can. And it will be the last time you will see me in our bedroom!" He is so nervous, he did not even catch my slur. We go into the bedroom, I tell him to let me see his cell phone and with hesitation, he hands it over. I scroll the numbers he has dialed, lord and behold he called her on the way home. Why? He tells me he was letting her know it was over and I knew everything. (He's smarter that I thought.) I go ballistic at this point, I scream, "YOU CAN'T EVEN COME HOME WITHOUT CALLING THAT SLUT!" He wants to explain. He still has no idea about the tape. (He calls himself a good cop.)

I tell him a few months ago, I was giving his daughter a bath and she asks me a question. "Why does daddy have a girlfriend?" I tell her, "Daddy has girls that are friends, that's all, honey." I told him that night when he came in from work, and he laughed. We both did. Kids can say the darnedest things! I did not forget it. Would you? No, No, No!

I tell him "listen" and I turn the tape on. Tears rolled down his face and he tells me, "We just talked, nothing happened!" RIGHT! He is on his knees, crying and begging me to forgive him. I cry, but stand firm. I tell him I have NO trust in you, marriage is a trust issue and YOU have lost mine. He keeps telling me, "It's not what you think. PLEASE!"

I already have his clothes in garbage bags on the porch, and he loads them in the patrol car, and leaves. I cry all night long. My mom and dad try and help me through my hurt. TIME is all that will help.

Later that night, I feel guilty. Why you ask. Because I've

got no idea where he had to go. His family does not live close. A friend of OURS calls and tells me he is there with him and his family, and he is torn up over this. I feel guilty because he is so upset. Stupid. I'm the one that is hurt. I'm just glad my days off are Saturday and Sunday. As soon as the weekend passes, I'm sitting in my lawyer's office early Monday morning.

My lawyer, also a friend, asks me "are you sure you want to jump into a divorce?" I'm looking at him with tears and turn on the tape. I cry again while listening to it with him. I can't believe this is happening to me. My husband was so supportive while I was sick, now I wonder if it was all a lie. I wonder if my whole marriage was a BIG FAT LIE? My lawyer, after listening to the tape, asks, "What do you want?" I want a divorce! I explained it like this...my mind is not a VCR (DVD's weren't a big thing then); there is not an erase mode in our brains, just replay! He understood loud and clear. He had never thought of it like that. He tells me to come back in a few days and all the paperwork will be ready for me to look over.

I walk out of his office and who is sitting in a truck waiting on me, her boyfriend. (He is also supposed to be one of my husband's friends). He wants to know if the rumors are true. "What rumors?" I ask. He looks at me with tears and confusion; I know what he's asking. I tell him I have the tape, but he really should not hurt himself by listening to it. He keeps insisting and I keep trying to discourage him. I give in. This is about the fifth time I've listened to the tape, I just get silent and numb when I hear it. We put the tape in his tape player in the truck. I tell him to be prepared because it's a lot of hurtful things about him too. He tells me he has to know. I really did not want to hurt him; one person hurting is enough, (Me)!

He begins listening to the horror! I look at him and he

has his head on the steering wheel, crying. (Men also cry mule tears, amazing, huh?) I try to console him, why I don't know. Heck I need consoling too, but I feel so sorry for him. He finishes the tape and looks at me and says "Thank you."

Thank you for what, hurting you? I get out of his truck, and he leaves.

I go home and my husband is sitting on my patio with the dogs. (GO FIGURE). I think that's where he needs to be at this time, with the dogs. He still doesn't get that when I heard the tape, every bit of air that I was breathing was knocked out of me. He tells me we need to talk. I can't think of anything to say but cut downs and ugly words. He tells me he does not know why he TALKED to her, still swearing he did not sleep with her. He says he has made an appointment with a friend of his that is a marriage counselor. That is when I tell him, I filed for a divorce. He starts begging me, just don't do it. Please! I reply, "I told you if you ever cheated on me what would happen, remember?"

I tell him to turn the table around, what would he do? All he can do is cry. Then of course I cry. There is no doubt he made a mistake, but right now, I can't help him. I can't forgive and forget. I've been a very weak person, but right now, I stand strong! All I've been through mentally and health-wise seems to have made me a strong woman at this point in my life. I'm proud of myself, actually! I know you're thinking, what does this have to do with knowing your body? A lot, like how strong minded you are, how you know if you can heal your broken heart and understand your emotions. I know what some of you are thinking, "How can I be so cold?" I'm not; I've got a big, soft heart. I know in time I'll forgive him, but this is just hard for me to do right now.

We get divorced! Being such a good person, wanting to

help him figure out why he did this to US, I agree to start going to the counselor with him. He has been going for several weeks, but his counselor asks him to see if I would come to help him work out why he did this. When I agreed, the deal is separate cars, but if he does not listen to EVERYTHING I've got to say, I'll quit! He agrees.

I drive 30 miles one way every week, sometimes twice a week, to meet with him and the counselor. The first couple of times, my anger would over-ride everything else. The counselor told him it's only right to hear all my anger and hurt. The least he can do is take it, since he dished it out. After six months of this, I realize that he had also helped me come to terms with not only my ex's issues but also my health issues. So this is one time I figured maybe this was a good thing, not the cheating, but the counseling! I was told I did not need to come anymore, but my ex continued and then just quit. I can't answer why.

During all of this we continued to keep a professional working relationship. We did try to work things out after the divorce; we just could not get over the hump. To this day we still work together and I'm his boss.

We are even best friends; he will always have a very special place in my heart and soul.

Later that year...(yes, there was more to the year than just the above) my mom and I go on a well deserved vacation to Florida. We're on the beach, which is a good place to be when vacationing and my mom said something about my chest looking funny. I told her it's just because she hadn't seen me in a bathing suit since the surgery. We vacationed for nine wonderful tanning days and flew back home. I called my surgeon because my implant does look like it has moved up higher than the other. I go to see him and you will never believe what happened...my implant which is tear-shaped has turned upside-down. Crazy!!! Now, this isn't a big emergency so there is no big hurry for surgery. I'll just look funny, well, think about it. I've got a bald teardrop boob to begin with, now I have an upside-down bald teardrop boob. Unbelievable right? I thought so too. I'm divorced, pretty tanned in all the right places and, all things considered I think I look pretty good strutting up and down the beach in my bikini, and this whole time I've got an upside-down bald-headed boob. My surgeon has a conference in China, so we wait until he returns before we schedule. This is where I believe God takes care of me...

It's a good thing he decided to wait until after his trip to China, because while I am awaiting his return to have the implant fixed something I never thought would happen, did. I became pregnant!! Gotcha!!! Just kidding!

I was taking a bath and as most women do who have had breast surgery I do a breast exam on the left side (remember the right side is upside-down and just skin and implant) and you will not believe what I found. I was sitting in the tub and to my horror my nipple had blood and green coming out of it. Yeah, you're reading this right. I pray I'm wrong with my thinking.

I call my mom, again, crying, again. She tells me to call my boss, tell him what's going on and drive down to her house so we can go to my general surgeon (my doctor that had done the mastectomy). I call my boss (he's one of my best friends) and tell him what is going on. He tells me to call him as soon as I know anything, to not worry about work. So I pack my clothes, get my dogs and off to Mother's house we go. She lives about an hour from me, but closer to my doctors.

The whole time I'm driving I pray the nightmare is not starting over. How many times can Humpty-Dumpty be put back together? If the worse happens, what man will ever want me (I know, I know)? I've got an appointment the next day (Thursday) to see what my fate will be. I feel really, really alone, even though I've got my family. I feel myself pulling into a shell again. I tell myself, "You are strong, you can handle whatever life throws your way!" God brought me this far, he'll bring even farther.

I know life throws a lot of curve balls, but really I've hit the world series of curve balls. (No trophies or million dollar contracts either.) The next morning Mom and I get ready and go to my doctor. I don't get signed in before I'm called back to the exam room. The nurse gives me the blue and white stripe robe and tells me she (the doctor) will be in to see me in a few minutes. That's just what it was, a few minutes and she walks in the room. She does my exam, mammogram, and takes a culture of the fluid coming out of my nipple. She tells me she will be right back. Thirty minutes pass and I'm wondering out loud to mom, what is she doing? To my surprise she comes back in "with" the pathology report. She had gone to pathology and waited on my results. I'm telling you she is a wonderful doctor! She looks at me, a little sadness in her eyes, and begins, "we're lucky we have caught this early." I'm thinking caught what early? She continues, "we'll do a radical mastectomy, clean up and start over like before." She tells me she will notify my plastic surgeon and that she will go ahead and remove the upside-down implant while I'm asleep. Dazed and confused, I agree and she goes out of the room while I collect my thoughts and composure. She comes back a few minutes later and tells me surgery is schedule the next day. WOW! She isn't wasting any time.

I don't believe I opened my mouth on the way back to my mom and stepdad's house. I don't even know if I blinked. I thought I was having that nightmare! Bet you think there is no way one woman can go through all of this and survive. Well, I'm writing this and you're reading it, right? I'm living proof, and I know it's all because of my faith, family and friends.

Morning comes quick. It's still dark outside. Last night I called my dad and told him there wasn't any sense in him coming because I will need him later (to take me to start reconstruction). He wasn't real crazy about my idea but went along with it. I know his heart was breaking as well as mine. He knows Mom is there and will take care of me. Mom and I get to the hospital, check in and go to my room. I know the routine all too well. Just get it over with. I come out of surgery with the stinky drainage tubes and bulb again. No breast, my implant removed. Talk about FLAT CHESTED! I thought the pain was excruciating the first time; one side was all I had to deal with, now I'm dealing with both sides cut wide open. Both of my armpits are throbbing, every part of my body is hurting. The circulation stockings are cutting the blood supply off to my brain. (At least they felt like it.) So much for wearing a bathing suit the rest of the summer. A pre-adolescent girl has more to put in a top than I do. But, if I've learned anything, I'm still beautiful, but boobless! I'm really okay with all of this. Used to it? Maybe. Glad to still be alive? Absolutely! Do I like the stinky drainage tubes? Absolutely not! What are seven to ten days worth? Just a thing! This is the attitude my second time around with mastectomies.

The drainage is a lot worse this time, 60 to 100 cc's a day. Not good. I go back to the doctor to get my stitches out, but the tube has to stay. I told her it stinks (the smell of the fluid) she tells me if she removes it too soon, I'll get a bad infection. So I deal with it. As long as I have her drainage tube (not mine, I would never take credit for that thing) I have to go back and forth to see her every five days. This goes on for 45 days. She takes "her" drainage tube out on the 45th day. I hated to see the drainage tube leave, we'd become such good friends, and I had almost grown attached to it. (Funny, hah hah!) This was a big relief. The drainage tube actually was a pain in the butt (okay, okay, it really wasn't in my butt, I know). I'm finally home free, right? Wrong! Several days later, my chest (left side) started filling up with fluid, looks like my breast is growing back. Not! I started to run a high fever. I call her (my doctor's) office and she meets my dad and me PDQ. (Pretty darn quick) I felt terrible. My head hurt, my chest hurt and the fever had me really dragging. I ask my dad to go in the exam room with me; he had already seen the good, bad and ugly. He is the one who helped me with the drainage tubes for so long after I came home from Mom's. She tells us she will have to drain the fluid off. Well, guess what is used to drain stuff off the body? The needle was huge but I'm too sick to care. Wrong! When she put that needle into my sore, flat chest, I thought I was going to faint. She pulled 50cc's of fluid off. She tells us to watch it (fluid build up in a flat chest ain't real hard to see) and if it happens again get in touch with her PDQ. She bandages me up and we drive home. Dad goes and gets my antibiotics (Yes, the pharmacist sends me Christmas cards) for the infection. A few days pass and it happens all over again, soooooo, back to the doctor's we go for my chest to be emptied, drained (gosh, now I know what draining a lake or pond must involve). (Reconstruction you get fill ups, remember) every time the fluid was pulled out, my fever would go down to almost normal. When my chest would fill up (not in the good way) my fever would go up. This went on for about the next three or four weeks.

I know as long as this was happening, reconstruction

surgery on both sides would be impossible. So I began wearing the bra the American Cancer Society people brought me after the first surgery. I can't remember exactly where I was but, while out one day, someone came up to me and told me my prosthesis had slipped out of the bra and was coming out the top of my shirt. Instead of being embarrassed, I fell out laughing. I couldn't stop laughing. I think it had to be one of the most hilarious moments of my life. Maybe it's not that funny to you, but it was very funny to me at the time. Maybe I just finally see the humor in all of what I've been through. I'm happy just to hear myself laugh again.

Six months have passed and finally I can go and see my plastic surgeon. I know what to expect. I also know I don't want the teardrop implants, no duhhhh, huh. My only concern at this point is, what about nipples? How do they make them and where does it come from? How long do I have to wait after all the other surgery before I can have them? Would nipples be worth the pain? These are all questions I have absolutely no clue about. My doctor tells me we can worry about all of that later. We are facing about a year of reconstruction. So it begins, AGAIN!!!

The expanders are put in and the painful filling and stretching of the skin begins. I thought I had forgotten how bad it hurt, but am well reminded when I come out of surgery. Today I wonder sometimes if the Tram Flap would not have been easier. I talked to a lady that had had the Flap procedure and she says she would never ever do it again. She tells me she would definitely have implants. So I know I've made the right decision, for me anyway. I notice, during the expander period, that my left armpit is really deep, kind of like a cave or something. It doesn't look full like my right armpit. On my next appointment for a fill up (ding, ding, hey, do you remember when you use to go to a gas station for a "fill up" and you drove your car over this black cord on the ground and it went...., ok, am I telling my age?) I bring this to my doctor's attention. He tells me he will try and fix it when we take out the expanders and put in the final implants. He then does the fill up and while I'm lying on the table, he asks about me joining this study about people with new implants. I want to know if it will help other women and he told me he hoped so. That's all I had to hear. I will do any thing to keep someone else from having to go through any part of what I have gone through. Silicone implants were not even discussed when I had the first reconstruction. I guess all the controversies you hear about on the news make doctors leery of silicone.

I know women who have silicone and those who have saline implants. My opinion, the silicone implants look more natural. This is only an opinion (everyone has one) and my first implant was saline. It wasn't soft (like a real breast) but it wasn't what I call hard either. The implants my doctor is offering for the study are silicone with a rough texture outside. The first one I had was smooth on the outside. The rougher edge (outside) is supposed to cut down on scar tissue build-up. I'll have to go see him often for the study, but I look at it this way, maybe I can help just one woman and then my job is complete, and I helped him with his study.

As soon as the expanders could be removed, the study starts and I receive the new implants. My doctor will try to fix my left underarm while he's stuffing the rest of my chest. I never thought to ask, what if these turn upside-down until the day of my surgery. He chuckled, no, I think he laughed out loud and finally said that it will be all right because they're round (get it, upside-down, right-side up, it won't matter! I smiled at him, and off to sleep I went. Being put to sleep is what I hate the most about surgery because you can't control anything about it. Nothing!

After surgery I feel like a two-ton truck has parked itself on my chest, both sides were just throbbing. Again the ice packs become a dear friend. The armpit is fixed and I'm really happy about this. It was so hard to shave under my arm with a big cave-in. Now it will be so much easier. I really couldn't say how many times I've cut myself before he fixed it.

As far as my new breasts are concerned, when the bandages come off, I know they will be beautiful with or without a nipple. I know it sounds crazy, I'm happy, because I feel since I'm in the medical study maybe God has a reason for all of this. I learned a long time ago, God never puts more on us than we can handle (He DOES however, push the limits).

I feel like I've won the lottery because I paid attention to my breast and I caught things really early. That is how I can share my story with you. After all of the pain goes away, I'll get my nipples put on to make the surgery complete.

I discuss having my nipples put on with my family first (can you imagine starting that conversation?). Mom says go for it, my brother tells me whatever decision I make he will be there, my dad, well, let's just say he is old school and thinks that it is unnecessary (thinking about surgery, etc., I suppose) and my step-dad is supportive about whatever I decide to do. My brother talks to our dad, who is 69 yrs old, and explains to him that it's a big part of the reconstruction and if he had some type of "male" surgery he would want his finished too.

So I make the appointment to discuss the procedure with my doctor. I'm in shock with what I hear. Here it goes...my doctor comes in the room with paper to draw how this is done. I call them nipples and he calls them the areola. He explains they will be non-functional. What this means is no sensation to anything, not even cold weather. Understand, when you have a mastectomy you lose a lot of feeling anyway, all the cutting, I suppose. Some areas of both my so-called breast are numb to the touch, but I do have what they call "phantom pains."

Let me explain. Even without my nipples, sometimes if I get chilled it feels like they come to attention. (Like headlights.) As far as my breasts are concerned, sometimes it feels like they are asleep. (Like when your foot or arm goes to sleep.) Then at times they feel like they are itching, and nothing I do stops the itching. I can't imagine how people who have lost a limb honestly put up with phantom pains. Mine really don't hurt; it is just aggravating. It's really hard to explain how they feel, but I tried.

Now, back to how they can build my nipples. One way is this: they can take tissue from the inside of my vagina (once again, I think a man came up with this idea). I can hear it now, if and when I meet a man, fall in love, I tell him my vagina is on my breast. OOOOH GROSS! That is NOT what I would want to tell someone, and you know as well as I do men are curious and I wouldn't lie about it. One thing I know about myself is, if you don't want to know something, don't ask!

The second choice of where a nipple can be retrieved is…. from the hipbone area. This sounds better than having them made from my VAGINA! I guess I'm still amazed that anyone would want her vagina on the breast area. Aren't you? You all know which way I chose, hipbone!!!!

Now I wonder how in the world they are going to make a nipple out of my hipbone. Well, believe it or not it CAN be done. I've got to decide several things. One is how much I want the nipple to stand out? What color do I want them to be? How round do I want the area around the actual nipple?

Decisions…decisions!! I never knew how much of an artist

a plastic surgeon has to be. The only difference is they don't sign their work. (At least I don't see a signature!) I tell him I want them to have small headlights, not real dark (pinkish), the round part about the size of a quarter. (Not to be confused with looking like I paid a quarter for them!)

He laughs, he sort of thinks I'm crazy! (Meaning a great outlook on life, not psycho!!) I've just finally decided that life is thrown at you. Deal with it!

We arrange all the surgery stuff yet again. My dad takes me to have this done. I am told to be at the surgery center at six o'clock A.M.!! We only live an hour away, but dad tells me to be ready at four o'clock in the morning. We leave at four and are sitting in the parking lot of the surgery center (in his unmarked patrol car as he is the chief of the sheriff's department) because the surgery center isn't open yet. A police car pulls up and asks what are we doing sitting there in the parking lot? My dad tells him that we are there for my surgery. Get this...I'm in a pair of nice pajamas with a robe and house shoes on. What did the man think...we were the pajama robbers???? Always wear something comfortable when you have surgery. It isn't like when you wake up and get to go home you are going to feel like going out to Red Lobster or anything! It's about a quarter to six and we finally see a light come on in the center. I tell him to go and check the door, but it's still dark and the door is still locked. (That is why they give you certain times to be there! You think?) All I want is a cup of coffee, but I couldn't have anything to eat or drink after midnight the night before. Finally about ten after six we can go into the building. You will never believe what the first thing I smell is...COFFEE! Is that mean or what? Now I'm thinking, call me back already, this is torture, because I love coffee.

The nurse comes out and calls me back; my dad kisses me

on the cheek and tells me he loves me. Even though I'm over 40, I'm still daddy's little girl and he is a sweetheart. But see I'm lucky, I've got two dads that love me because my stepfather treats me like a daughter too. So I guess you can tell I may be a little spoiled (to those who know me, I SAID A LITTLE). My doctor comes in with his FAMOUS MAGIC MARKER and starts drawing on my two bald heads so he can center the nipples and make them even with each other. See, I told you they are artists.

Same routines, I go to the operating room and the nurses prep me. Except this time, where do they put the blood pressure cuff? Well I'll tell you, believe it or not they put it on my thigh. Remember when you've had a mastectomy do NOT let them take the blood pressure on the side you had your surgery on. There's always another way to get your vital signs. You know the drill is to count backwards from 100, so I make them happy and count to I think 98 or 97. Sweet Dreams, again!! While I was asleep, I had a dream (okay, a nightmare) that when I woke up my nipples were huge (they were the size of quarters, not the areola) and they cut them from my vagina and didn't shave my hair. How gross is that?? A huge hairy nipple from my vagina (yep, I'm gonna be popular with the boys). I can't remember ever dreaming before or maybe I did. I don't remember, I was asleep!

So when I wake up, the first thing I do is feel (okay, grope) my vagina area, whewwww, I'm safe there! Thank goodness. The dream really seemed real; it was in color and everything! Of course the doctor has me bandaged up so I can't see my nipples, so I start asking the nurses how big they are. No one knew and my doctor had already left to go to the hospital for rounds. The nurse tells me I can remove my bandages in two days and shower only, no bath. I was proud not to have the drainage tubes; I can deal with the rest.

Two days have passed; the pain is not really bad except my hipbones hurt and burn. (This is because of the nerves being cut and blood vessels being moved to my breast area). I can tell you this; it is probably one of the easiest surgeries I've been through. I get up that morning, my mom is with me and we go to the bathroom to remove the bandages. I'm really not afraid to look this time. I'm actually rather excited (emotionally, thank you very much, for you smart asses out there). This is the beginning of the end!

I feel my heart racing from excitement and anticipation while we remove the bandages. It takes us a few minutes to get them off, they are really stuck on and we don't want to pull the nipples off (I know that sounded strange but, I met a woman who was taking her bath and she looked in the water and her nipple was floating in the tub). So we were being very, very careful. I look in the mirror and they look black and huge, I freaked! They look awful. I call my doctor and his nurse tells me that it's normal after surgery. The black is bruising and scabs, the protruding nipples will go way down in time. I felt so relieved; I thought I really had some big headlights!!! She also tells me the color will fade and I will have to be tattooed (now I've heard of nipple rings, but not nipple tattooing) after I heal. I ask her will that hurt? She tells me, well, not really. What is not really? I've never had a tattoo, so I don't really even know what they do. So I'll have to wait until I heal, and I don't like the unknown! At this moment I'm happy my nipples aren't going to poke someone's eye out! Just kidding!

Remember, my mom is at my house a lot during all this and we are both real pet lovers so, to protect me from her puppies and the way they love to jump on you, she puts up a puppy gate to block off the hallway going to my bedroom.

Well, also down this hallway is my bathroom and on this particular day, I've got to go to the potty. Well, as I'm stepping over the gate I fall flat on my face, well my chest (with these sized boobs, my face is safe, if you catch my drift). I look up and she is running full bore to me. I told her I'm okay, just look around and see if my nipples are on the floor. They weren't, so that had to mean they were still on my chest. Finally, I get a break! Now I just hope I haven't jarred them to where they'll come off in the tub. Well, good news. My nipples stayed on while I bathed and after! Great huh?

I heal and go to have the tattooing done (thank God a specialist wasn't called in for this or I'd had the biker guy from a Hell's Angel club image going through my head the whole time). But this part is all new to me. The nurse comes in and puts numbing crème on the areola area and tells me this will help lessen the stinging from the needles. Understand I have gotten to know this office staff really well, to the point of friendship actually. I look at her like she is crazy. No one said anything about more needles. She explains that the needles help put the color down into the skin. She shows me several colors of ink (OMG, color swatches for nipples, I've heard it all) to make up my mind on the color. I feel like I'm building a woman like in the movie "Weird Science." Have any of you seen that movie? The only difference is I don't have a male sitting at the computer helping with all the other parts. So she tells me if I don't like any of the colors she has brought in we can mix them to the color I want (am I the only one here feeling like I'm in Wal-Mart having paint mixed for a bedroom?). I tell her I just do NOT want them dark, because I never wear a bra. I don't want them to show (color) through my tops. I choose a pretty pinkish color. Baby pink is my favorite color, so we get the color close to a dark baby pink. She tells me we are ready for putting the color on each nipple. The ink is applied directly to the skin, and then she takes a round-looking object with a lot of very small needles and pushes the color into the skin. The needles really are not hurting me; I think it is more the sound the machine makes (kind of like the dentist office). It is amazing how it pushes the ink into my skin and the color comes to light, like the color of a nipple. (I didn't even have to put my vagina skin there, thank goodness, yuck!!!)

It made the area bleed a little, but the whole experience was so interesting and so amazing to see how far science has come for women like me. I had a great-aunt that had a mastectomy and as a child I can remember if someone knocked on her door she would tell them to wait while she took her titty out of one pocket and her teeth out of the other. She was so funny! She never had the options I had. So I'm really glad I DO NOT have to tote my tits in my pocket. I guess if I did, if a man wanted to play with my breast, I could just take them out of my pocket and hand them to him! Just kidding!!!!!

Now in all seriousness:

I never realized how many women are going through the treatment of breast cancer. The realization of this is most of them have never been sick until the breast cancer has taken hold. I had to realize, there is absolutely nothing I could have done to change what has happened (breast-wise). So I have to make the best of a bad situation. I'm still here, still on this earth for a reason, maybe it's just to help one of you. I know I carry on a lot of crap, kidding around and such, but breast cancer, ovarian cancer, heck; just any type of cancer is serious. The outlook YOU have going into whatever treatment you have been offered is the BIGGEST part of your healing and wellness. Your hair will grow back! You will stop getting sick at your stomach from chemo. And the stronger you are (mentally), the more you can deal with what's in front (sorry, no pun, really) of you. Always, always, have a higher power in your life. PAY ATTENTION TO THE CHANGES IN YOUR BODY. DO NOT IGNORE THE CHANGES, BIG OR small! It could make all the difference. Let me explain:

Some one I loved very much died of lung cancer last year. She was like a mother to me. She also worked for me. Anyway, she ignored a lot of signs her body was telling her before she finally broke down and went to the doctor. When she did go, they told her she had cancer. She comes to my house. We sit down and talk for hours. I tell her, "WE can beat this." She tells me the doctor recommends high doses of chemo and radiation. Her sons live a long way from here, so my ex (I told you we were still friends) and I take the responsibility of getting her back and forth for her treatments. He takes her for radiation and I take her for her chemo. She has a friend come to cut her hair short before it starts falling out and one of her sons would fly in as much as he could. Her eldest son, toward the end, stayed with her. She had a bad stroke and lost the use of the whole left side of her body. She was the type who hated depending on others. She was always really independent and vivacious in life. We lost the fight on August 24, 2004. I miss her so very much. If she had listened to her body and gone on to the doctor, maybe (oh, just the possibility of maybe) she could have been with us for many, many more years.

I had another friend, who was very young (late 20's) who passed away a couple of years before she did. He always complained of heartburn. His mom and dad are very dear to me to this day. Every time I saw him he was eating some type of antacid. I kept telling him to go to the doctor; he kept saying, "I just ate something that didn't agree with me." Late one afternoon in August, I answer the 911 line and it's his dad on the other end saying he thinks his son is dead. I handle the call while he is on the phone. Once we hang up I lose my entire composure, call my ex (he was also working) and we go to their house. His brother, mom and dad were sitting in the living room when we walked in. I felt like I had lost my little brother. We embraced with lots of crying. The autopsy report stated the vessels to his heart were very small, and even if he had been in the hospital when it happened he probably would not have survived.

My aunt had never been sick a day in her life. She was only in the hospital when she had her children (six) and we all were very close. They would come from New Mexico every summer and stay at our house. I get a call from her oldest daughter (we are VERY close) and she tells me, "Mother has brain cancer." I'm in disbelief. A couple of days later, my mom and I drive to New Mexico to see her. When we arrive she has undergone her first brain surgery and the doctors tell us the type of cancer she has is very aggressive. She begins chemo and radiation almost immediately. They removed as much of the tumor as possible but the tumor would grow so fast. Did she have signs which she ignored? I don't know. She lost her battle right after Christmas four years later. I believe she had a strong will to live, which is why we had her as long as we did.

I have other stories, but I don't want to bore you. These are just very dear to my heart. Listen to your body, please!

I'm doing pretty great in my life now. I still have the lupus and other problems. My friend and doctor (she takes care of me), well, we are working together and my medication is working. She keeps a very close eye on my problems as well. I take notice of any changes and tell her, regardless of how minor they may seem. I've been seeing her for about 15 years.

She knows me better than I probably know myself. As far as the study with my plastic surgeon goes, I'm still in it. If I call either office, they know me by my first name. Some of them even recognize my voice before I give my name.

I'm happy, still not married. I have wonderful family and friends. I have two beautiful dogs. A black Shar-pei named Demi and a little Fiest named Molly. All of my friends, who have children or are having a child, always share their joy of motherhood with me. I continue to work for E-911; I'm the supervisor now. My ex-husband still works for me and we are very close friends. He has re-married now (No, not to her). Now he is going through a divorce. This time it is not his fault. My boss, well, let's just say he is the greatest boss and the best friend a girl could have (and he's a man, can you believe it). He has been very understanding concerning all my surgeries, as have been my board members. My church has been great, always bringing food and prayers (not necessarily in that order) while I was down.

My biggest worries about myself now are that I'm getting older. I worry about getting wrinkles on my forehead, (I do not worry about drooping boobs) and bags under my eyes. But the greatest thing is that I'm still here so I believe that I need to just get some great face cream!

I know some of the humor in this may be a little corny, but if you cannot laugh at some bad situations you will go crazy. Laughter is the best medication. Just remember this one thing: we, as women, cannot change what has happened or what is happening to our bodies, so what we have to do is make the best of a bad thing. We are all beautiful in our own way! Never think you aren't, because you are. I had to learn this lesson the hard way.

For those of you who are going through anything close to

this and you are married, let your husband be there for you. I didn't for a long time and I paid the consequences.

Maybe this will even help men understand what you are going through, so let him read it and you talk to each other after both of you read this. I know in my heart it will only bring you closer.

I don't have a lot, just what I've told you. I pay my bills. I have a car payment. I guess what I'm telling you is, "I'm just an average person who has to work for a living." It is important to me to share my story with others. All I pray is that someday my story may help someone else cope with what she believes is the absolute worst thing in the world happening to her. Life is granted us and it's up to us to decide what to do with it. So, don't go through life always thinking your cup is half empty, it's really half full and it's up to us to fill it up the rest of the way.

To all service men and women, thanks for all you do to keep the United States safe and free!!!!!!!!!!!!! Also I dedicate this book to all of those who I have lost and touched my life in so many ways.

GOD BLESSES YOU ALL AND MY PRAYERS ARE WITH EACH AND EVERY ONE OF YOU.